MIND-GUT CONNECTION DIET

FOR NOVICES

Enriched Recipes, Foods, Meal Plan & Procedures That Focuses On Brain And Gut Health, Immune Response, Easy Digestion And More

DR. MATEO GABRIEL

DISCLAIMER

The information in this book is only meant to be used for general reading. In any way, the author and publisher do not promise or represent that the information in this work is full, correct, reliable, appropriate, or available. This includes any warranties that are expressed or implied. Because of this, you should only rely on this material at your own risk.

This book is not meant to replace professional help. If you have any questions about a subject, you should always get help from a qualified expert. The author and distributor of this book are not responsible for how the information in it is used or abused.

The author's thoughts and feelings are shown in this book. They do not necessarily represent the official policy or stance of any other person, group, employer, or business.

Any third-party material that you can get to through this book is not endorsed or backed by the author or publisher.

The information in this book is correct at the time it was published, after all possible checks. However, the author and distributor are not responsible for any loss, damage, or inconvenience that may be caused by mistakes or omissions.

TABLE OF CONTENTS

CHAPTER ONE 10

INTRODUCTION TO MIND-GUT CONNECTION DIET..10

RECOGNIZING THE LINK BETWEEN MIND AND GUT
....10

THE MIND-GUT CONNECTION'S SIGNIFICANCE 13

THE PATH TO BETTER MENTAL AND DIGESTIVE ...14

CHAPTER TWO 16

THE MIND-GUT CONNECTION'S BASIS.....................16

EXAMINING THE AXIS BETWEEN BRAIN AND GUT16

PHYSIOLOGY AND ANATOMY 17

BRAIN-BASED COMMUNICATION 18

THE GUT MICROBIOTA'S FUNCTION 19

CONTENTS OF THE GUT MICROBIOME 20

CHAPTER THREE...22

MICROBIOME AND EMOTIONAL STATE....................22

TRANSMITTERS AND HORMONES.........................22

FEELINGS AND SEROTONIN.................................24

CHAPTER FOUR 28

KNOWLEDGE OF THE MIND-GUT DIET.....................28

THE MIND-GUT CONNECTION DIET'S BASICS 28

FOOD SELECTIONS 29

BALANCE OF NUTRIENTS 30

THE TIME OF MEALS 31

CHAPTER FIVE 34

DIETARY ITEMS THAT AFFECT THE MIND-GUT
RELATIONSHIP...34

RICH IN PROBIOTIC FOODS 34

DIETARY PREBIOTICS............................35

FOODS THAT REDUCE INFLAMMATION 36

CHAPTER SIX 38

THE MIND-GUT RELATIONSHIP AND MENTAL
WELLBEING 38

SADNESS AND NERVOUSNESS 38

DIET AND MENTAL HEALTH ARE LINKED...............39

SUCCESS STORIES AND CASE STUDIES 40

MENTAL WELL-BEING AND BRAIN STRUCTURE 41

STOPPING COGNITIVE DETERIORATION 42

CHAPTER SEVEN.....................................44

DIGESTIVE HEALTH AND PHYSICAL FITNESS 44

INTESTINAL HEALTH...............................44

TAKING CARE OF TYPICAL DIGESTIVE PROBLEMS.45

RESTORING THE GUT'S CORTEX 46

IMMUNE SYSTEM ASSISTANCE 47

THE IMMUNITY AND GUT HEALTH 48

MEALS TO BOOST YOUR IMMUNE SYSTEM 49

CHAPTER EIGHT 52

REALISTIC IMPLEMENTATION STRATEGIES...............52

MEAL PREPARATION 52

MAKING WELL-COMPOSED MEALS 53

MINDFUL DINING METHODS 54

COMBINING EXERCISE 54

FITNESS AND DIGESTIVE HEALTH.........................55

BENEFITS OF THE MIND-GUT DIET IN TANDEM....56

OVERCOMING OBSTACLES...................................57

MANAGING YOUR CRAVINGS 57

CHAPTER NINE 60

MEAL IDEAS AND RECIPES 60

MORNING MEAL 60

LUNCHTIME...61

SUPPER...63

GUT-HEALTHY SMOOTHIE BOWLS 64

GUT-NOURISHING SALADS.................................66

BALANCED LUNCHES FOR ENERGY 67

MIND-GUT CONNECTION DINNER RECIPES 69

COMFORTING AND NUTRIENT-DENSE DINNERS...70

CHAPTER TEN 72

SUSTAINABLE LIFESTYLE CHANGES 72

MAKING THE MIND-GUT DIET A HABIT..................72

ADJUSTING FOR DIFFERENT LIFE STAGES 74

STAYING INFORMED ON GUT HEALTH..................76

CHAPTER ONE

INTRODUCTION TO MIND-GUT CONNECTION DIET

RECOGNIZING THE LINK BETWEEN MIND AND GUT

In recent years, there has been a growing awareness of the complicated relationship that exists between the gut and the mind, revealing a deeper level of interaction than just digestion. Often called the "Mind-Gut Connection," this link represents the reciprocal exchange of information between the central nervous system and the enteric nervous system, which is located in the gastrointestinal tract. Emerging research indicates that the gut is crucial in regulating mental and emotional well-being, going beyond the traditional concept of the stomach's role in nutrient absorption and waste removal.

Examining the Mind-Gut Connection in greater detail reveals that a network of neurological, hormonal, and immunological processes are involved in this symbiotic interaction. Neurotransmitters, a wide range of biological signaling molecules, and the vagus nerve facilitate the complex communication between the gut and the brain. Given the interdependence of gastrointestinal and mental health, this dynamic connection serves as the cornerstone of a holistic approach to health.

The importance of this interaction about eating habits is one of the main topics of understanding the Mind-Gut Connection. In addition to providing our bodies with nourishment, the food we eat has a significant impact on the microbiota in our guts, which in turn affects the synthesis of hormones and neurotransmitters that control mood and cognition. Often called the "second brain," the stomach serves as a central controller for several physiological functions, highlighting the vital role it plays in preserving general health.

THE MIND-GUT CONNECTION'S SIGNIFICANCE FOR DIET

Beyond the realm of conventional nutrition knowledge, the Mind-Gut Connection holds great significance in eating. It clarifies how food decisions can either exacerbate or lessen mental health conditions like sadness and anxiety. A diverse population of bacteria living in the digestive tract, the gut microbiota is crucial for the production of vital vitamins, the breakdown of complex carbohydrates, and immune system modulation. Thus, the makeup of the gut microbiota directly affects brain activity and emotional stability, underscoring the significant influence of nutrition on gut and mental health.

THE PATH TO BETTER MENTAL AND DIGESTIVE HEALTH

Starting the path to a healthier gut and mind requires a multimodal strategy that incorporates dietary adjustments, mindfulness exercises, and lifestyle changes. Understanding the connection between gastrointestinal and mental health encourages people to take a holistic approach, realizing that taking care of one always takes care of the other. Along with practices that enhance mental health, this journey calls for a diligent effort to build a balanced and healthy diet that supports the gut microbiota.

The Mind-Gut Connection is an intriguing nexus between holistic health, nutrition, and neuroscience. Comprehending the complex interplay between the mind and the stomach presents prospects for interventions that beyond conventional medical limitations. A holistic approach that takes into account the symbiotic interaction between these two key systems is necessary to achieve a healthy mind and stomach. This will help to promote a state of homeostasis that is essential to general well-being.

CHAPTER TWO

THE MIND-GUT CONNECTION'S BASIS

EXAMINING THE AXIS BETWEEN BRAIN AND GUT

The complex interaction of communication and influence between the brain and the stomach, also known as the "brain-gut axis," is reflected in the delicate relationship between these two essential systems. A network of neuronal, hormonal, and immunological circuits that together control several physiological processes are involved in this reciprocal communication. The brain-gut axis affects not only digestive processes but also emotional and mental states, and it is essential for preserving homeostasis. Deciphering the workings of this relationship is essential to understanding the mysteries surrounding both gastrointestinal and mental health.

PHYSIOLOGY AND ANATOMY

The anatomical and functional characteristics of the brain and digestive system are covered in the anatomy and physiology of the brain-gut axis. The enteric nervous system (ENS), a sophisticated network of neurons implanted in the lining of the stomach, is in communication with the central nervous system (CNS), which is made up of the brain and spinal cord. The vagus nerve and other brain circuits facilitate this communication, which enables the real-time coordination of digestive functions. The immunological and endocrine systems also have a role in controlling gut function, highlighting the complex relationship between the brain and gut.

BRAIN-BASED COMMUNICATION

A complex interaction between neurotransmitters and neuropeptides underpins neural transmission in the brain-gut axis. The transmission of impulses between the brain and the gut is facilitated by neurotransmitters such as gamma-aminobutyric acid (GABA), dopamine, and serotonin. These neurotransmitters' modulation affects mood management, the body's reaction to stress, and cognitive performance in general. Gaining knowledge of the neurological communication pathways can help us understand how stress and emotional states might affect gastrointestinal health and vice versa.

THE GUT MICROBIOTA'S FUNCTION

The function of the gut microbiota is a topic of growing study about the brain-gut relationship. The gastrointestinal system is home to billions of microorganisms known as the gut microbiota, which includes bacteria, viruses, and fungi. These microbes actively take part in the synthesis of bioactive chemicals, immunological regulation, and nutrition metabolism. The dynamic interaction between the gut microbiota and the host organism affects systemic functions, such as those about the brain and mental health, in addition to local gut health.

CONTENTS OF THE GUT MICROBIOME

The particular kinds and quantity of microbes that are present in the gastrointestinal system are referred to as the gut microbiome's composition. A healthy symbiotic relationship with the host depends on the diversity and balance of the gut microbiome. Numerous elements, including nutrition, way of life, and exposure to the environment, might influence the gut microbiome's makeup. Many medical illnesses, including gastrointestinal disorders and mental health problems, have been linked to an imbalance known as dysbiosis. Examining the complex interplay between the composition of the gut microbiota and the brain-gut axis presents opportunities for therapeutic approaches meant to support overall health.

CHAPTER THREE

MICROBIOME AND EMOTIONAL STATE

TRANSMITTERS AND HORMONES

Numerous variables contribute to the complicated interplay between the microbiome and mental health, with hormones and neurotransmitters being key players. The gut-brain axis affects both physical and mental health by acting as a bidirectional communication channel between the central nervous system and the gastrointestinal tract. Hormone and neurotransmitter regulation is one of the essential components of this communication.

Cortisol and insulin are two important hormones that regulate stress and metabolism, respectively. These hormones are produced and regulated in part by the gut flora, which affects metabolic processes and stress reactions. An imbalance in the composition of the microbiota may cause dysregulation of hormone levels, which in turn may lead to mental health issues such as sadness and anxiety.

Mood regulation is mostly dependent on neurotransmitters, which are chemical messengers that let nerve cells communicate with one another. Known as the "feel-good" neurotransmitter, serotonin is especially significant when it comes to mental wellness. The gut produces most of the body's serotonin, and the microbiota affects how it is synthesized there. Changes in the makeup of gut microbes can affect serotonin levels, which may result in mood disorders.

FEELINGS AND SEROTONIN

Serotonin's capacity to affect pleasure and well-being is closely related to its function in mood regulation. Through the fermentation of dietary fibers, which results in the creation of short-chain fatty acids (SCFAs), the gut microbiota contributes to the production of serotonin.

Consequently, the expression of genes involved in serotonin production is influenced by SCFAs. As a result, abnormalities in the gut microbial ecology may contribute to mood disorders by cascade effects on serotonin synthesis.

Moreover, the vagus nerve, a key nerve that connects the gut and the brain, is involved in the bidirectional communication along the gut-brain axis. The vagus nerve's activity and the subsequent release of neurotransmitters like serotonin are both influenced by the microbiota. This complex interaction emphasizes how crucial a diversified and well-balanced gut flora is for mental health.

Research on probiotics with mental health benefits, or "psychobiotics," has shown how the gut microbiota may be the target of therapeutic interventions that might improve mood and lessen the symptoms of mental illnesses. Probiotics may affect the synthesis and control of hormones and neurotransmitters, such as serotonin, by altering the microbiota.

A complex web of interactions underlies the link between microbiota and mental health, with hormones and neurotransmitters playing a major part. Gaining knowledge of how the gut microbiota affects serotonin production and regulation opens up important possibilities for mental health therapy.

The discipline of psychobiotics, which is still in its infancy, has the potential to produce innovative methods for treating mental health conditions by influencing the gut-brain axis.

CHAPTER FOUR

KNOWLEDGE OF THE MIND-GUT DIET

THE MIND-GUT CONNECTION DIET'S BASICS

The foundation of the Mind-Gut Connection Diet is the knowledge that there is a close relationship between the health of the mind and the gut and that eating habits have a significant impact on preserving this delicate balance. The tenets of this diet emphasize the symbiotic relationship that exists between the brain and the gut, acknowledging that mental health is influenced by gut health and vice versa.

FOOD SELECTIONS

A fundamental component of the Mind-Gut Connection Diet is food selection. Consuming a wide variety of whole, nutrient-dense foods that support the gut microbiota is the main focus. Including a range of fruits, vegetables, whole grains, and lean proteins is part of this. meals high in probiotics, such as yogurt and fermented meals, are also recommended to support the growth of good bacteria in the gut. People can improve their general state of well-being by selecting foods that feed their bodies and minds.

BALANCE OF NUTRIENTS

Another important idea in the Mind-Gut Connection Diet is nutritional balance. A balanced intake of vital elements, such as carbs, proteins, fats, vitamins, and minerals, is emphasized in the diet. Reaching this equilibrium is thought to maintain the complex communication system between the brain and the stomach. Because of their possible benefits for cognition, the intake of good fats—like the omega-3 fatty acids found in fish and nuts—is especially important. Maintaining a healthy nutritional balance is essential for maintaining mental and emotional stability in addition to supporting physical health.

THE TIME OF MEALS

The Mind-Gut Connection Diet views meal timing as an important component in addition to food selection and nutrient balance. The method recognizes the importance of circadian rhythms and how they affect many body processes, including digestion. It is believed that eating meals at regular intervals that correspond with the body's natural cycles can improve nutritional absorption and aid indigestion. The goal of this deliberate meal planning strategy is to align the gut-brain axis, which will enhance communication between these two essential systems and improve general health.

The three main tenets of the Mind-Gut Connection Diet are thoughtful food selection, nutrient balance, and thoughtful meal planning. Through these concepts, people hope to enhance their mental and physical health by cultivating a healthy relationship between the gut and the mind. This all-encompassing method emphasizes the relationship between eating patterns and mental well-being, encouraging a way of living that nourishes the body and the mind.

CHAPTER FIVE

DIETARY ITEMS THAT AFFECT THE MIND-GUT RELATIONSHIP

RICH IN PROBIOTIC FOODS

Foods high in probiotics are essential for fostering the mind-gut connection, which is a network of communication that runs both ways between the brain and the digestive system. When ingested in sufficient quantities, probiotics—live microorganisms, mostly beneficial bacteria—offer health advantages. By encouraging the growth of helpful bacteria and inhibiting the growth of harmful ones, these foods help maintain a healthy gut microbiota. Fermented foods such as kefir, sauerkraut, kimchi, and yogurt are high in probiotics and help maintain a healthy gut flora.

DIETARY PREBIOTICS

Prebiotic foods work hand in hand with probiotics to support a healthy gut microbiota. Prebiotics are indigestible fibers that feed the good bacteria in the stomach. Prebiotics support a varied and robust gut microbiota by encouraging the development and activity of these microorganisms. Prebiotic-rich foods include onions, garlic, bananas, and asparagus. By adding these foods to the diet, one can foster the growth of advantageous bacteria and, in turn, have a good impact on the mind-gut axis.

FOODS THAT REDUCE INFLAMMATION

Beyond microbial balance, the influence of nutrition on the mind-gut link also takes into account the function of anti-inflammatory substances. Anxiety and depression are among the mental health conditions for which chronic intestinal inflammation has been connected. Eating foods low in inflammation helps reduce this inflammation, which leads to a healthy gut and, in turn, a more balanced mind. Turmeric, berries, leafy greens, and fatty fish are a few foods that have anti-inflammatory qualities. These products have ingredients that support general gut health, lower inflammation, and regulate the immune system.

A symbiotic relationship between the mind and gut can only be fostered by recognizing the complex interactions that occur between the gut and the brain and include a range of probiotic-rich, prebiotic, and anti-inflammatory foods in one's diet. This integrative approach to diet promotes a harmonious balance in the complex communication network between the gut and the brain, which benefits mental health in addition to digestive health.

CHAPTER SIX

THE MIND-GUT RELATIONSHIP AND MENTAL WELLBEING

SADNESS AND NERVOUSNESS

The complex interrelationship between the gut and the mind has drawn more attention recently, especially in light of its consequences for mental health. More and more people are viewing anxiety and depression—two common mental health conditions—through the mind-gut relationship. Studies indicate that mood regulation and emotional well-being are significantly influenced by the gut-brain communication that is enabled by the gut bacteria. Anxiety and depression have been linked to dysbiosis in the gut microbiota, underscoring the reciprocal relationship between the mind and stomach.

DIET AND MENTAL HEALTH ARE LINKED

Grasp and utilizing the mind-gut link requires a grasp of the relationship between nutrition and mental health. Our mental and emotional moods are significantly impacted by the food we eat, in addition to our physical health. Dietary habits that are high in omega-3 fatty acids, probiotics, and prebiotics have been associated with a decreased risk of mental health problems. On the other hand, diets heavy in sugar and processed foods have been linked to a higher risk of developing anxiety and depression. The notion of "food as medicine" is becoming more and more popular, highlighting the part that nutrition plays in promoting mental health.

SUCCESS STORIES AND CASE STUDIES

Examining case studies and success stories provides insightful information about how to use the mind-gut connection in real-world situations. People who have changed their lifestyles to support gut health or who have adopted diets that are favorable to the gut frequently report feeling better mentally. These tales highlight the potential benefits of gut microbiome-focused customized therapies for mental health outcomes. These instances add to the increasing amount of data that supports the theory that treating gut health issues can enhance traditional mental health therapies.

MENTAL WELL-BEING AND BRAIN STRUCTURE

The mind-gut relationship is mostly dependent on brain health and cognitive function. According to recent studies, gut bacteria may contribute to neurodegenerative disorders and have an impact on cognitive functions. The gut-brain axis, which is the term for the bidirectional communication between the gut and the brain, is made up of intricate signaling channels that affect cognitive performance. Modulating the gut microbiome through dietary modifications or probiotic administration is one strategy to improve memory and focus.

STOPPING COGNITIVE DETERIORATION

In light of the mind-gut relationship, preventing cognitive decline is an important factor to take into account. Preserving cognitive health is becoming increasingly important on a global scale as the population ages. Research on the gut microbiota's role in age-related cognitive impairment is ongoing. Lifestyle choices that promote gut health, such as exercise and diet, may help maintain cognitive resilience as we age. Developing preventive measures against cognitive decline presents a promising opportunity when the mind-gut relationship is comprehended and utilized.

There are numerous implications of the mind-gut relationship for mental health, including food, anxiety and depression, cognitive performance, and the prevention of cognitive decline.

CHAPTER SEVEN

DIGESTIVE HEALTH AND PHYSICAL FITNESS

INTESTINAL HEALTH

Maintaining general physical well-being is greatly influenced by digestive health. Our digestive system is in charge of processing food, drawing nutrients out of it, and getting rid of waste. The digestive system makes a substantial contribution to the general health and vigor of the body when it operates at its best. Preventing more serious health consequences and promoting well-being require addressing common intestinal difficulties.

TAKING CARE OF TYPICAL DIGESTIVE PROBLEMS

Common digestive issues including gas, indigestion, bloating, and constipation affect a lot of people. Many times, food decisions, stress, or underlying medical ailments are to blame for these problems. Some of these typical digestive discomforts can be relieved by eating a well-balanced, nutrient-rich diet high in fiber. In addition, stress management methods, mindful eating, and drinking enough water can all support improved digestive health.

RESTORING THE GUT'S CORTEX

Promoting general well-being requires, among other things, healing the gut lining. One of the most important defenses against dangerous drugs entering the bloodstream is the intestinal barrier, or the lining of the stomach. Poor food choices, long-term stress, and using specific drugs are some of the factors that might damage the integrity of the gut lining. Consuming gut-healing meals including collagen-rich foods, fermented foods, and bone broth can help repair the gut lining and enhance digestive function.

IMMUNE SYSTEM ASSISTANCE

It is commonly known that immunity and gut health are related. A large percentage of the immune system of the body resides in the gut. The diverse population of bacteria and other microorganisms that make up a healthy gut microbiome aids in the body's defense processes and aids in the prevention of illnesses. Probiotics help support a healthy balance of gut bacteria and improve immunological function. They can be found in fermented foods and supplements.

THE IMMUNITY AND GUT HEALTH

Maintaining general physical well-being as well as preventing infections depends on immune system support. The immune system is mostly supported by the gut, and the body's capacity to fight off infections is enhanced by a healthy digestive system. The body's immunological response can be further boosted by adding immune-boosting foods, such as vitamin- and antioxidant-rich fruits and vegetables, to the diet in addition to probiotics.

MEALS TO BOOST YOUR IMMUNE SYSTEM

Foods high in nutrients provide a wide range of choices for those with robust immune systems. Citrus fruits, strawberries, and bell peppers are good sources of vitamin C, which is well known for strengthening the immune system. Foods high in zinc, another vitamin crucial to immune system function, include nuts, seeds, and lean meats. Incorporating green tea, garlic, ginger, and turmeric into the diet can also give beneficial chemicals that boost immunological function.

Sustaining a robust and healthy body requires a grasp of the complex relationship between gut health and physical well-being. Through the treatment of common digestive disorders, repair of the gut lining, and bolstering the immune system via appropriate nutrition, people can improve their general well-being and vigor. Developing a conscious, well-balanced lifestyle and diet is essential to support good gut health and, by extension, a solid basis for physical well-being.

CHAPTER EIGHT

REALISTIC IMPLEMENTATION STRATEGIES

MEAL PREPARATION

Meal planning is essential to leading a healthy lifestyle because it enables people to intentionally choose their daily dietary intake. The procedure entails carefully weighing nutritional requirements, preferences, and objectives. One can guarantee a well-rounded, balanced diet that satisfies nutritional needs by organizing meals in advance. This tactic promotes self-control over eating patterns and helps one steer clear of impulsive meal selections.

MAKING WELL-COMPOSED MEALS

Meal planning and creating balanced meals go hand in hand. To guarantee a varied range of nutrients, several food groups are incorporated. For general health, it is important to maintain a balance between macronutrients like proteins, fats, and carbs and micronutrients like vitamins and minerals. This methodology not only bolsters physical health but also helps maintain consistent energy levels all day.

MINDFUL DINING METHODS

People are encouraged to be completely present and involved in the dining experience by using mindful eating techniques. This entails observing signs of hunger and fullness, enjoying the tastes and textures of food, and putting away other distractions when eating. A more positive relationship with food is fostered by mindful eating, which also improves digestion and reduces overindulgence.

COMBINING EXERCISE

Exercise is a crucial part of a comprehensive strategy for good health. Frequent exercise not only helps with weight management but also strengthens mood, promotes general well-being, and improves cardiovascular health. To make fitness a long-lasting component of a person's routine, it's critical to select workouts that complement personal tastes and objectives.

FITNESS AND DIGESTIVE HEALTH

Physical activity has a good impact on the microbial makeup and diversity in the gut, which is why there is a connection between gut health and exercise. Frequent exercise has been associated with a more robust and diversified gut flora, which is important for immune system function, nutrition absorption, and digestion. This emphasizes how crucial it is to take a holistic approach to health that incorporates both dietary decisions and physical activity.

BENEFITS OF THE MIND-GUT DIET IN TANDEM

The complex interaction between the stomach and the mind is acknowledged in Synergies with the Mind-stomach Diet. The Mind-stomach Diet, which takes into account the two-way connection between the stomach and the brain, emphasizes how dietary decisions affect mental health. A person can achieve optimal mental and digestive health by combining mindfulness techniques with food.

OVERCOMING OBSTACLES

Overcoming Obstacles is a crucial component of any journey centered around health. Social situations can be difficult since they frequently entail activities centered around eating. Making educated decisions, expressing dietary preferences, and planning ahead of time can all help you manage social situations without sacrificing your health objectives.

MANAGING YOUR CRAVINGS

Managing Cravings calls for a thoughtful, balanced strategy. Rather than seeing desires as roadblocks, people should look into better substitutes that both satiate their cravings and support their nutritional objectives. Being aware of the physiological or emotional triggers behind cravings enables people to make deliberate decisions and keep a sustainable, well-balanced eating pattern.

Doable tactics for execution cover a range of lifestyle facets, such as meal preparation, healthy eating, exercise, mindful eating, and handling obstacles including social settings and temptations.

CHAPTER NINE

MEAL IDEAS AND RECIPES

MORNING MEAL

A hearty breakfast sets the stage for a healthy day in advance. A well-liked and delectable choice is Gut-Healthy Smoothie Bowls. A range of fruits, vegetables, and other healthful items are usually blended into a smooth, creamy consistency and served in these bowls. Common ingredients like oats, kefir, and yogurt improve digestive health in addition to improving the texture of the bowl. These ingredients promote healthy digestion since they are high in fiber, prebiotics, and vital nutrients.

Checking out Probiotic-Rich Breakfast Options is a great alternative for breakfast. Probiotics can improve the balance of intestinal bacteria and support a healthy digestive tract when added to breakfast. Fermented fruits, yogurt, and kefir are delicious additions to breakfast. These high-probiotic foods support healthy gut flora, which is essential for general well-being.

LUNCHTIME

Gut-nourishing salads are a delightful noon meal that also happens to be good for your gut. These salads have a variety of fruits, nuts, and vegetables in addition to the standard greens. Including foods high in fiber, such as beans, broccoli, and leafy greens, can aid in digestion and give you a feeling of fullness. Incorporating an assortment of vibrant veggies not only improves the appearance but also guarantees a wide range of nutrients.

Eating a balanced lunch is crucial to sustaining focus and productivity throughout the day. A combination of complex carbohydrates, healthy fats, and protein make up a well-balanced meal. When combined with whole grains and a range of vegetables, foods like grilled chicken or tofu offer sustained energy and help avoid the mid-afternoon energy slump.

Adding nutrient-dense meals to your lunch helps healthy gut function and general well-being.

SUPPER

The Mind-Gut Connection Dinner Recipes highlight the complex relationship that exists between the gut and the mind. These recipes highlight foods that are good for the digestive system and promote mental health. Crucial ingredients include leafy greens, whole grains, and fatty fish high in omega-3 fatty acids. These ingredients not only promote gut health but also contribute to cognitive function, making for a well-rounded and mindful dinner experience.

Comforting and Nutrient-Dense Dinners round off the day on a satisfying note. These dinners prioritize wholesome ingredients that provide a sense of comfort without compromising nutritional value. Root vegetables, lean proteins, and whole grains are often featured in these recipes, offering a mix of essential nutrients. Warm soups, stews, or roasted dishes can be both soothing and nourishing, creating a perfect end to the day that supports overall health and well-being.

GUT-HEALTHY SMOOTHIE BOWLS

Smoothie bowls have become a popular and delicious way to promote gut health while providing a refreshing and satisfying meal. These nutrient-packed bowls typically include a base of blended fruits and vegetables, often combined with yogurt or a dairy-free alternative. Ingredients such as berries, bananas, kale, and probiotic-rich yogurt contribute to a diverse array of nutrients that support a healthy gut microbiome. Adding ingredients like chia seeds, flaxseeds, or nuts enhances the fiber content, promoting digestive regularity and overall gut well-being. Topping the bowl with fresh fruits, granola, and a drizzle of honey not only adds texture and flavor but also introduces additional vitamins and minerals that contribute to a balanced and gut-friendly meal.

GUT-NOURISHING SALADS

Salads can be a powerhouse for gut nourishment when thoughtfully composed with a variety of colorful and fiber-rich ingredients. Incorporating leafy greens like spinach, kale, or arugula provides essential vitamins and minerals, while vegetables such as tomatoes, cucumbers, and bell peppers contribute prebiotic fibers that fuel beneficial gut bacteria.

Adding fermented foods like sauerkraut or kimchi introduces probiotics, further supporting gut health. Including a source of lean protein, such as grilled chicken or tofu, not only enhances the salad's nutritional profile but also provides amino acids crucial for overall well-being. Dressing the salad with olive oil, which contains healthy fats, can aid in the absorption of fat-soluble vitamins and contribute to a balanced and gut-nourishing meal.

BALANCED LUNCHES FOR ENERGY

Creating balanced lunches that sustain energy levels throughout the day involves combining a variety of macronutrients and micronutrients. Incorporating complex carbohydrates like whole grains, such as quinoa or brown rice, provides a steady release of energy. Pairing carbohydrates with lean proteins like fish, beans, or poultry helps maintain satiety and supports muscle function. Including a colorful array of vegetables not only adds vitamins and minerals but also introduces fiber that aids in digestion. Healthy fats, found in sources like avocados or nuts, contribute to a feeling of fullness and support nutrient absorption. Crafting a balanced lunch not only fuels the body but also helps maintain focus and productivity by preventing energy crashes.

MIND-GUT CONNECTION DINNER RECIPES

The mind-gut connection is a fascinating aspect of overall well-being, highlighting the intricate relationship between mental health and gut function. Dinner recipes that prioritize this connection often include ingredients that support both physical and mental health. Fatty fish, rich in omega-3 fatty acids, contribute to brain health while also providing essential nutrients for the gut. Whole grains, such as barley or quinoa, contain fiber that supports gut bacteria and may positively impact mood. Additionally, incorporating colorful vegetables and herbs not only enhances the visual appeal of the meal but also introduces antioxidants that promote overall health. Mindful eating practices, such as savoring each bite and minimizing distractions, further strengthen the mind-gut connection and contribute to a holistic approach to well-being.

COMFORTING AND NUTRIENT-DENSE DINNERS

Comforting dinners can still be nutrient-dense by selecting wholesome ingredients that nourish the body. Root vegetables like sweet potatoes or carrots add a comforting and hearty element while providing essential vitamins and fiber. Lean proteins, such as turkey or lean beef, contribute to muscle health and satiety. Incorporating legumes like lentils or chickpeas not only adds texture but also introduces plant-based protein and fiber. Using whole grains, such as whole wheat pasta or quinoa, enhances the meal's nutritional profile. Including a variety of herbs and spices not only elevates the flavor but also provides additional health benefits. Comforting and nutrient-dense dinners offer a satisfying way to end the day, providing the body with essential nutrients for overall well-being.

CHAPTER TEN

SUSTAINABLE LIFESTYLE CHANGES

MAKING THE MIND-GUT DIET A HABIT

Embracing a sustainable lifestyle involves not only addressing external practices but also fostering internal well-being. The Mind-Gut Diet, a concept rooted in the intricate connection between the mind and the gut, underscores the significance of a holistic approach to health. This dietary regimen recognizes the bidirectional communication between the brain and the gastrointestinal system, emphasizing the impact of food choices on mental and physical well-being.

Incorporating the Mind-Gut Diet into one's daily routine requires a shift in mindset and dietary preferences. This involves choosing nutrient-dense, whole foods that promote a healthy gut microbiome. Probiotic-rich foods such as yogurt, kefir, and fermented vegetables play a crucial role in supporting gut health. Additionally, the diet encourages the consumption of prebiotics, found in fiber-rich foods like fruits, vegetables, and whole grains, which fuel the growth of beneficial gut bacteria.

Developing the Mind-Gut Diet as a habit necessitates mindfulness in eating practices. Mindful eating involves savoring each bite, being attuned to hunger and fullness cues, and appreciating the sensory experience of meals. By making mindful eating a regular practice, individuals can establish a deeper connection between their mental and digestive well-being, creating a sustainable foundation for a healthier lifestyle.

ADJUSTING FOR DIFFERENT LIFE STAGES

Sustainability in lifestyle changes is inherently linked to adaptability, especially when navigating different life stages. Life is dynamic, and the factors influencing dietary choices and overall well-being evolve with age, personal circumstances, and external responsibilities. Recognizing this, individuals seeking sustainable lifestyle changes must tailor their approaches to accommodate the specific needs and challenges associated with different life stages.

For instance, young adults may focus on establishing healthy habits that contribute to long-term well-being, while those in midlife might need to address changing metabolism and hormonal fluctuations. Parenthood introduces a new set of challenges, requiring adjustments to accommodate family needs and priorities. As individuals enter their senior years, considerations may shift towards nutrient absorption, bone health, and maintaining cognitive function.

Sustainable lifestyle changes demand a nuanced understanding of individual needs at various life stages. Flexibility and a willingness to adapt to evolving circumstances become paramount, ensuring that health goals remain realistic and achievable across the diverse phases of life.

STAYING INFORMED ON GUT HEALTH

An integral aspect of a sustainable lifestyle is staying informed on the latest developments in gut health. The field of gut microbiome research has expanded significantly, revealing the profound impact of the trillions of microorganisms residing in the digestive tract on overall health. To foster a sustainable lifestyle, individuals must prioritize ongoing education and awareness about the factors influencing gut health.

Staying informed on gut health involves keeping abreast of scientific studies, emerging trends, and expert recommendations. Regularly updating knowledge about the connection between gut health and various aspects of well-being, such as immunity, mental health, and metabolism, empowers individuals to make informed decisions about their dietary choices and lifestyle practices.

Incorporating reputable sources of information, consulting healthcare professionals, and participating in community discussions on gut health contribute to a well-rounded understanding of this complex and evolving field. By staying informed, individuals can make conscious, evidence-based choices that support not only their digestive systems but also their overall health and longevity, thus embodying a sustainable and informed approach to well-being.